A Journal for Karen

by

Peggy L. Chapin

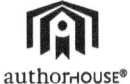

authorHOUSE®

AuthorHouse™
1663 Liberty Drive, Suite 200
Bloomington, IN 47403
www.authorhouse.com
Phone: 1-800-839-8640

First published by AuthorHouse   2/5/2008

Printed in the United States of America
Bloomington, Indiana
This book is printed on acid-free paper.

ISBN: 978-1-4343-5236-1 (sc)

Library of Congress Control Number: 2007908873

The Holy Bible, King James Version, The World Publishing Company, Cleveland and New York

Ecclesiastes 3:1-8

To everything, there is a season, and a time for every purpose under heaven:
A time to be born, and a time to die;
A time to plant, and a time to pluck up what is planted;
A time to kill, and a time to heal;
A time to break down, and a time to build up;
A time to weep, and a time to laugh;
A time to mourn, and a time to dance;
A time to cast away stones, and a time to gather stones together;
A time to embrace, and a time to refrain from embracing;
A time to get, and time to lose;
A time to keep, and a time to cast away;
A time to rend, and a time to sew;
A time to keep silence, and a time to speak;
A time to love, and a time to hate;
A time of war, and a time of peace.

From me, Peggy, to my family:

I feel I must share the following with not only you, but also others. I hope I have not overstepped my boundaries, as I sometimes have been known to do. Karen reminded me of it many times over the years, but she did tell me recently that I have improved. I loved my sister dearly. Now, there is a void in my life. There is a bond between sisters that words cannot explain. It is just there—even now.

The following pages were taken and adapted from a journal I kept for Karen. She was to receive this journal when the cancer was gone, to help her remember and fill in the gaps of her life during the months of illness where memory had been suppressed. It then became a way to cope with the events of this dreaded disease. Although each of you have your own special memories, this journal has become a way for me to remember Karen's last few months through a sister's perspective.

May you each receive comfort in my thoughts and know it is (1) because of my love for my sister and each of you that I share, *A Journal for Karen*, and (2) that by doing so it will, in some way, help others.

*K*aren Kay Price was born in 1953, the second daughter of Elmer and Betty Zabokrtsky. She had an older sister, Peggy, who was born in 1951, and a brother, Keith, would join the family in 1956. She graduated from Washington High School, Washington, Kansas, in 1971 and received an associate degree from Cloud County Community College, Concordia, Kansas, in 1991. She married Bill Acree in 1973. She loved her children; family was everything to Karen. She gave birth to three sons: Aaron, Caleb, and Luke. She remarried in 2001 to Ken Price and became stepmother to Cindy, Kristi, and Craig. She loved her grandchildren. Every one of them was special to her. She treated her sons-in-law and daughters-in-law, as they were her own.

Karen was a member of the United Methodist Church, PEO, United Methodist Women, Lions Club, and Modern Pioneers Club. She held offices in several of these organizations. She had been a club and project leader in 4-H. She loved to travel.

She loved flowers and enjoyed gardening. She loved animals. She was an animal caregiver, puppy coordinator, training instructor and then CEO of the Kansas Specialty Dog Services, now known as KSDS, Inc. Karen had a passion for her work and dedicated her life to helping others.

Karen was diagnosed with cancer in August 2006. She fought this dreadful disease with everything she had and then some, until at last, on January 25, 2007, the cancer took her from us.

Karen's spirit surrounds us.

Family and friends remember her smile, her laugh, her love, spiritedness, vision, wisdom, and courage.

She is deeply missed.

There is a void.

The objective of sharing *A Journal for Karen*, is to help make it possible for others who find themselves in the circumstance she did, to not only give them hope, but allow them to have the ability to survive and conquer their cancer.

I wrote a journal to Karen, my sister, while she was going through her cancer. I did this so she would be able to remember things that happened during her months of treatment. I planned to give this journal to Karen after her treatments were done and when she was on the road to recovery. Karen survived six months after being diagnosed. She was a fighter. She made a point to be positive, even when those around her found it difficult to do so. She never asked, "Why me?" but I did, many times. She said more than once, "I would not wish this on anyone."

For a variety of reasons, I have not included everything I wrote to Karen in her original journal. I have, however, chosen to share the following pages with you, the public, in order to:

(1) Promote positive where there is negative.
(2) Help fill a void that runs deep.

(3) Help comfort others who find themselves where we were during Karen's illness.

(4) Provide some humor along the way where little can be found.

(5) Help others receive treatment from the dreaded disease—cancer.

Karen was only fifty-three years of age when cancer invaded her life and took her from us. I remember her telling us there were less than 15,000 cases per year of her type of cancer. Therefore, research monies were just not as abundant as with other cancers—the ones we hear more about like breast cancer, colon cancer, and prostrate cancer. One obviously becomes more aware of the "other" cancers when it affects them personally.

All profits from this book will go toward research for finding the cause, treatment, and eradication of Large B-Cell Non-Hodgkin's Lymphoma of the brain.

August 6, 2006

Karen—I'm not sure why I am writing this journal. It may be more for me than you. I remember telling you I had a project for us to do. I asked you to call me whenever you had free time and we'd have coffee, go for a Coke, and start our project. Purses—felted. We would work on them only when we were together. You had purchased a couple of sergers and given me one of them earlier in the year. You told me it was up to me to find a project for us to do together. I've used the serger and looked for a "project" to use it for but decided since you love to knit, we'd do the purses instead. In addition, it would be a good excuse to get together. Seems we've not done that as much as we should lately since work, family, etc., always seemed to have taken precedence. (A typical response 99 percent of the world seems to also have in common with us.) Time is precious, and we tend to forget that.

I played at our church service on July 23, 2006. Instead of speaking to me afterwards as you always do, you just looked at me for quite some time. Then, you turned around and walked off—very unusual. I let it slide. The week went by. On July 28, 2006, the folks called to tell us Ken had taken you to see the doctor. They thought you might be on the verge of a breakdown—stress-related. I felt so guilty I hadn't noticed more or helped somehow in preventing it. How could I, your sister, not know that you needed me to be more aware of your situation?

Aaron had told me earlier (around July 19) that he was concerned about his mom—that you seemed to not be yourself—and he asked if I had noticed anything. No, I had responded—nothing major anyway, but I promised I would be more observant. You and Ken went to Salina for the weekend to rest, and to be free of obligations and work. You were scheduled for a CT scan. An abnormality showed up. Then, you had an MRI. Two abnormalities showed up. You had an appointment in Lincoln, Nebraska, with a neurosurgeon. You had a biopsy on August 4, 2006.

Waiting is difficult. I went to your home earlier in the week. We rolled (tried to roll) skeins of yarn. Two hours later, still on the same skein, I had finally completed mine. You keep cutting the yarn instead of straightening it. I finally took the scissors from you. The felting of yarn is forgiving, but too many short yarns probably are not a good idea. I finished the roll for you and gave it to you the next day. You seemed confused at times about what we were going to do with the yarn when it was in a ball, and where we would put it. You mentioned Grandma Guila several times. You knew you weren't right in your thoughts, but you really didn't know. You described it as being in a fog. You were easily distracted.

I wanted to go to Lincoln, but you and Ken had things under control and I knew you needed your space. Although against my will, I obliged and did not go. You stayed at Craig's and I knew you'd need me later. I didn't want to agitate you or upset you. Ken knew all he had to do was say the word and I'd be there. I gave you a hug and told you, "I love you." You said, "Thank you very much. That was nice of you to say." Keith and Caleb went to Lincoln anyway. Your biopsy went well. I called Ken and learned that you were getting along well. They were going to send you home Friday evening, and they did.

Saturday—no news about the biopsy. Ken says recovery from the procedure was good but you were having a bad day. I had gone to Kansas City for the weekend and when I got back on Sunday, I came to see you. You had been on the phone with Luke. Ken came to let you know I was there—three times. You were having trouble deciding what to wear and nothing seemed to fit. We had a nice visit. You seemed pretty good, but I could see a lost look in your eyes from time to time. We tried to pick plums but it started to rain—the first rain for weeks, and we welcomed it! I left and plan to return tomorrow to pick more plums and bring you both lunch. I'm off for the day and Mark has Rotary. You are scheduled to receive word in the morning about the biopsy. I pray it is benign. Everyone I talk to prays that it is benign. I can't think of any other result. I won't let myself think of anything but benign. I need my sis. I want her back. I promise to spend more time with you. I pray I get to.

August 7, 2006

The doctor's office called with the results. You had phoned me and sounded as if you would collapse. I brought you lunch and we talked for hours. Caleb came to see you. We picked more plums and made jam. It was the first time both of us had made plum jelly. Hope it works. We are occupying our time, planning a strategy, and realizing how we need to cope with what the future will bring. The folks came out to visit also. The clinic report gave lymphoma as the diagnosis. We do not yet know what kind. You are scheduled for an appointment Thursday to find out the particulars, and treatment, etc. It was difficult to hear but the treatments have improved so much. There are many calls regarding you. It was very hot and humid today and you were ready for a nap. We all left so you could rest better. You are to go to AA with Ken later tonight, and also you'll eat out.

August 8, 2006

We found out it is large B cell lymphoma of the brain. Everything I have researched about this condition says it is the best kind to have. It is the most treatable. We hope it has not spread. Many have called or e-mailed, including Mary Ann Crome, Mary Lou Walter, Nancy McCarty, and Rigs Brabec. Amy Kern, from Pennsylvania, sent an attachment regarding the mayor of Pittsburg who also has lymphoma. The article said that after one month of treatment, he will probably be able to resume a normal life again. He also had tumors of the brain—frontal lobe. He, however, has T not B. I spoke to Betty Kastl and Mary Alice Pacey. They said they had visited you. Christine Buchanan told me when Ken updated those at church about your health, it was the first time she'd ever cried in church during announcements.

August 10, 2006

Good news. At your neurosurgeon's appointment today, your stitches were removed and you were told this type of lymphoma usually doesn't spread to other areas of the body and is treatable. It is fast-growing and they will treat it aggressively. It's a long haul for you in the future, but the end results sound positive. I am so relieved and I know that prayers are still needed for you. I ate supper with you and Ken last night and I learned that you had a good day and were in good spirits. You had seen Aaron and his family the night before.

August 13, 2006

You made it to the family reunion around 12:30 p.m. You had gotten up at 5:00 a.m., and had breakfast with Luke in Oklahoma and then drove home. You didn't sleep at all. Ken said you didn't want to miss anything. You looked so tired, but upbeat. You spoke to so many people there. Ken took you home so you both could rest awhile. Your hands were shaking. I wonder if it is because you are tired or if it's the medication. You had a good weekend with Luke at Norman, Oklahoma. He saw the CD and films, and explained things to you. He and Ken took you shopping for a hat. Guess you saw a lot of hats, but you said you weren't ready for a hat yet. Luke also bought you a map so you could keep track of all those who were praying for you. What a great idea!

August 14, 2006

I called you after work and you had company. However, you said you were doing fine. Ruth Finlayson was here for her sister's surgery and then had come to see you. I know Dad had been out earlier but Mom had a terrible cold and didn't want you to end up with a cold, too.

August 15, 2006

Today you went to see Dr. Carlson—an oncologist in Manhattan. You'll be going back many times in the coming weeks. They want to make sure you have no cancer anywhere else in your body, and they want to make sure your heart can withstand the medicine. Hopefully, if all goes as planned, next Thursday will be your first day of treatment.

I talked to you on the phone. Ken had gone to a meeting for school bus drivers. I was going to come out, but Deb came over. She brought tomatoes for you, and she told me that you were tired and were going to bed shortly. I received an e-mail from James Lafevre regarding you. You are in his thoughts. Evelyn Fulton says you're on their prayer list, and the Popelka list of prayers. Todd Hynek says to tell Karen, "I wish her the best." He thinks a lot of both you and Ken. Have I mentioned the six-pack prayers? (Bert, Beth, Denise, Diane, Gayle, and me). Cindy Kongs sends prayers and is so good about sending cards. She has been in similar circumstances. Seems your class exchanges e-mails about you. How wonderful. In church on Sunday, they asked for continued prayers. I pray for you several times a day. Nancy Otott expresses concern. Steph and Evelyn have been super about you, me, and your family. Anytime I can drive or help, I will. Schedules are not in cement. I know I'm not mentioning everyone who asks about you—that would be just impossible, as there are so many. I will try to drop names every now and then to keep you updated on all those who are concerned about you. Names make it a little more personal. The doctor's office is always ready for any news we have to tell them. Of course, Mark, the kids and I are constants.

On a more humorous note—you can't believe how many people think you are "older" than me. If you'd color your hair that probably would solve that. You have beautiful white hair. I wonder what color it will be after treatments, but then, it really doesn't matter, does it?

August 16, 2006

You went to Manhattan for tests and will go back tomorrow—Thursday, for a bone marrow. You go Friday for a CT of your abdomen and chest. On Monday, they will put in a port-a-cath. You have a meeting next Thursday to find out the test results. You will most likely start chemo that day; probably five weeks of chemo one to three times per week, and then five weeks of radiation, five days per week. Betty Herda called the folks regarding you today. I also heard from several more people, including Carol Gray, and Tom and Sue Cooney. Deb gave you a cancer bracelet. She and Keith are going to Chicago for a couple days. The folks are going camping for the weekend at Fairbury. They went to Manhattan last weekend. Nate and Mark went on a golf outing for a couple days in Nebraska. Our thirty-fourth anniversary is Saturday. I think we're going to play golf and then go out to eat in either Manhattan or Junction City. The couples golf tournament will be held here on Sunday. Your medicine seems to be helping more. You seem more like Karen. You can hold conversations and keep on track. You must be exhausted. Ken has been wonderful. I'm sure he, too, is running on very little sleep.

August 21, 2006

You had your tests and are waiting to hear the results. The bone marrows were not fun. Diane Baskerville says you're on the prayer list at Afton. Also, the Cooney's have you on the Morganville Church prayer list. Arlene Hiesterman was asking about you. BJ Smart, Savages, and Watters also send regards. Don Imhoff is concerned. Think you have had a few good days and you have been able to go to a couple "fun" outings. You are having a pic-line put in today to help with chemo treatments. Hope that goes well. Golf tournaments, birthdays, anniversary, and school starting—busy schedules for everyone.

I purchased some gorgeous yarn, and will try to make you a hat for cooler weather. I hope it turns out. It's been a while since I have knitted—over thirty years. I'd better get in practice.

August 24, 2006

I spoke to Cindy Diehl. She was concerned and wanted to know about you. She suggested a particular cancer treatment center. She wasn't sure if you were in the hospital, or wanted calls. I gave her your phone number and she is going to call and give you the information. I thanked her for her support. You went to see your doctor today and we were all apprehensive, to say the least. Mom called while I was on the golf course for ladies night. You'd called and had good news—all testing showed no sign of cancer anywhere else in your body. Your treatments will start next Tuesday, August 29. You will have one treatment three times per week for four weeks—total of twelve weeks of chemo. There is a possibility that your tumors will be gone then. If so, you may not have to undergo radiation. Wonderful news! I'm so relieved. I'm excited for you and eager to pass on the news to others. Prayers and concerns are being answered.

Bob Neu asked about you. Golf mates of the night said "hello" and told you to hang in there. Connie Imhoff, Rigs Brabec, Jennifer Dague, Theresa Meyer, Gayle Monty, Laurel Navinsky, and Connie had also spoken to her sister Pat who sends best wishes and concern. My family are all so relieved and thankful. Keith will turn fifty on Saturday. There's a party at the lake but I'm on call. They will have to celebrate without Mark and I. It will be hard to top your gift of good news! It's been twenty days of roller coaster rides and you have about eighty-eight more to go before the end of your chemo treatment. Hang on. We'll be there with you during every step, bump, and curve. Your faith is strong and God is with you—the poem *Footprints* comes to mind.

August 27, 2006

I saw you Friday and you were in good spirits, clear minded, ready to begin chemo and be done with it. I don't blame you. You will be going to KU med center for treatment so you can be hospitalized while getting chemo in case they need to give counteracting drugs. The girls are hoping you'll stay over with them. It would make travel less tiring and they'd love to help somehow. Mark is golfing in a tournament today, and I'm trying to finish knitting a hat for you. Hope it comes out the way I want. It should help keep your head warm this winter, with or without a wig, if hair loss happens. Carol Gray made a statement to me in an e-mail that I've thought about for the last couple weeks. She said, "God sends us difficult times to let us know we can't do it without him." She should know as she's had her share of ups and downs in life. I consider her a very dear friend. She'll be a grandma for the first time this fall and is so excited about it.

September 4, 2006

Well, you've been in the KU Cancer Treatment Center since last Thursday—five days now—and I have no doubt you want to get home. At least you have one treatment down. The girls said they were so glad they went to see you. I'd spoken to you Saturday and again today. Guess there isn't a lot we can do to help your time go by any faster, except to let you know we're here for you. You'd had a different port-a-cath put in and finally got treatment started on Friday; the antidote was started on Saturday. Luke and Caleb were also there over the weekend. We'd all tried calling Friday but had the wrong phone number, and we'd also been given the wrong room number. Finally, we got it all straightened out. Mom and Dad had picked some peaches at your place and she was making a pie for you. I wish I could have a piece, too. We're going to Branson for a couple of days, then to a BBQ cook-off in Kansas City, golf/ shopping, and then back to work on Monday. We like the September vacations. September is cooler. It's usually crisp in the mornings, and the crowds are down.

Your birthday is coming up on September 10, and I hope you get to go to the baby shower for Craig and Andrea. Any type of crowd may not be good for your compromised immune system, but you also can't stay in a closet. We're still saying prayers in church for you. So many want to help, and what better way than prayer? God is with you. You will be a survivor. You have so much to give and so much yet to do. I am so looking forward to our aging together, whether gracefully or not. One treatment down, and seven to go. Lila Keesecker called and wanted an update. She sent well wishes.

September 13, 2006

Well, lots has been going on, and I need to catch up here. I had called and you were still at the KU cancer center on Tuesday, September 5, so I went to see you. You looked good but were soooooo ready to go home. I don't blame you. A room is just that—a room—white, no color, and you have a view of a brick wall. There is only so much you can read, and of course, there is TV to watch. You are coping with diabetes now due to the steroids. The staff has been good to you. Your doctor is honest and direct with you. It is difficult dealing with everything, but I truly believe your outcome will be good! Mark and I stayed a couple hours, and then we went to Rahe and Addie's for the night. Tomorrow we leave for Branson in the morning.

You're supposed to go home tomorrow. I called you on Saturday, September 9. You had already gone home on Wednesday morning and were doing well. It rained on the weekend but it was needed. You sounded good , and I learned that you will go to Lincoln on the 10th for the baby shower. Mark and I will play in the couple's tournament in Hebron on your birthday, so we'll see you on Monday, the 11th. You had a good birthday and went to work for the first time on the 11th. They had a birthday basket for you. You came home around 2-2:30 p.m., and felt good. I brought you the "hat" I made for you—it looks great on you, and it even fits! I'm so glad. The girls and I found a butterfly mobile and some battery candles for your KU room to help add color and a homey feeling, if that's possible. I hope it will give you a boost when you're away from home a few days during treatment.

You are going to Manhattan on Wednesday so they can correct the positioning of your port-a-cath. Then you go back to KU for your second treatment on Thursday. I saw Nina Meyer and she asked about you. She's had a double mastectomy and treatments at KU cancer center. She now has a year of treatment at KU, every three weeks. She wishes you well and maybe will see you sometime down there if your days coordinate. I am off today and have so much to do at home. I don't know where to start. It seems trivial in light of everything, but I do need to clean, do laundry, and putting some food in the fridge would be nice. You rolled your last ball of yarn at Mom's on Saturday night after she made you a birthday supper. I think I'll try to get mine done also, so we can get started on the purses. I had forgotten she had the yarn roller. Like you told her, you couldn't think straight so how were you to remember? I'm the one who should have remembered! Oh well, I've got to spend some extra time with you that way.

September 20, 2006

Well, you went last Thursday, September 14, and you're finally coming home today. You had many ups and downs during this trip. Diabetes is doing a number on you and your port needed adjusted. They are either reducing or eliminating your steroids and hopefully that will cause the diabetes to leave your system. I have no doubt it was rough. I called two or three times. You were very tired towards Monday. Ken's stay at the Hope Center seems to be going well. Not much news here. The kids are fine. Mark is cutting down the poison ivy tree! I'm so glad to be rid of that!! He plans to carve something out of the remaining wood.

I am waiting on your PRAYER QUILT to be passed to relatives and those who have yet to knot it. What a tremendous, moving, and heartfelt gesture. I'd never heard of it. Barb Wright sent it to Gracie and she's taken it to everyone you have an association with of some sort; it's been at church, Rotary, Lions, PEO, KSDS, and the hospital—to name a few. You should have some strong vibes and comfort coming from that quilt. You've touched many lives and everyone wants to give back. You are blessed. I so hope you feel better soon. Two down, and six to go. I'm getting over a slight cold, so it may be a couple days or so before I can see you. It must feel so good to be home. I know how it feels after a "fun" trip, so the treatment must make it more so. The folks are ready to see you. Dad's been working on the garage roof. Mom had a headache yesterday but rested and feels good today.

September 22, 2006

You worked the morning of September 21 and were a tad tired. You come in for blood work in the afternoon and stayed awhile for us to chat. It was so nice to get to talk to you. Your last session was a really tough one and I'm so glad it's over. Next week you go back. You're having an MRI Thursday morning and it will be compared to the first one. We're praying it shows improvement, and we don't even want to think about the reverse. You have some fluid around your heart, probably from the chemo. They're giving you twice the normal dosage, and they are being very aggressive. One of your nurses had the same diagnosis five years ago—that's a good statistic for you!

One of your doctors spent the entire night with you Monday and another was also there a lot. You were having chest pains and they had to unplug the port-a-cath. There seems to be a very caring, and supportive staff at the center. You mentioned a resident who was looking for a rural area and thought you would talk to Dr. Hodgson regarding talking to him about coming to our area. One of the doctors remembered Luke from his stint at KU—the physician is now on staff there.

Your hair is falling out. That doesn't bother you—finding hair everywhere does. Ken had given you a trim and vacuum. You had a couple of headaches. We're thinking that is a good sign, and means that the chemo is working. You aren't angry. You don't wish this on anyone. You haven't asked "why me?" You are anxious about what's next—the unknown. You cry, but a lot less than I would. You do extremely well. I can't imagine going through what you are. I wish, with all my heart, you didn't have to bear this horrible disease and its side effects. It seems so unfair—unfair to many. You may not ask why you, but I do.

Luke would like to be here with you, but you want him to continue his work so he can finish his doctorate. Caleb is able to come more often as his job schedule is more flexible than Aaron's or Luke's. Each of your boys has their own way of handling the fact their mom is not healthy. Moms are never sick. Moms help everyone. Moms make things better. Moms are always there. Give yourself a few months. I have no doubt in my mind that you will be on top of the game again. You will beat this horrible thing we know as "cancer." You will be a survivor. You will be. Prayers and God's blessings are with you.

Be strong. Do not let down your guard. Be positive. We are. We have to be strong in order to conquer this demon. Love conquers all, and Karen, there are all kinds of love around you—watch it conquer.

September 23, 2006

We worked on placing pins on the map to indicate the places where you have received cards from, and we only have a few left to do. The map is on the wall, and it is amazing to see the range of people across the United States whom you have heard from! Could you have ever imagined you'd touch so many people nationwide? The cards keep coming.

We did a few dishes and stuff to help get the house picked up. I really need to do mine, too. Isn't it unbelievable what just two people can accumulate and the mess we can make? How did we keep up when the kids were all home? You're in good spirits and getting along really well. Diabetes seems to be behaving better, but it is a long time to wait for MRI comparisons. It is next Thursday, but we are thinking positive!

September 27, 2006

We planted flowers—iris and daffodils. We look forward to seeing them come up in the spring. You're getting ready to go back to Kansas City. You have a huge week coming up.

September 28, 2006

Great news! Tumors are half the size, chemo is working, and everyone is so excited. However, you do have some blood clots in your legs and lung. They are taking some blood samples to see what else is going on. You're at the right place for treatment. What positive news—long way to go yet, but you'll get there!

October 1, 2006

I went to see you. Due to clots, you are only to get out of bed when you use the bathroom. You also had some positive growth in your blood cultures. They are not sure where the infection is but they are giving you antibiotics. The doctors decided you'd do better to be on oxygen. After being on oxygen for a while, and since the medicine is starting to kick in, you said you could already tell a difference! Your chemo is scheduled for Monday and the stress test was delayed. That's okay, since a couple extra days in KC will get you better. Between the pills, blood draws, oxygen checks, pain meds, etc., how do you get any rest?

Ken found Walmart! He went twice Saturday morning. We had lunch from the cafeteria, which was so good and we ate too much. You enjoyed my fruit! You had the prayer quilt on your bed and the butterflies were hung up. The medical staff seems nice. Addie called. She and Rahe are coming to see you later in the week. Luke called. He was at a seminar, but wanted to be elsewhere. He had had a bit too much coffee, so he was keyed up. It was so good to see you. You had a good attitude, and can see a positive outcome. Prayers are being answered. I left around 5:00 p.m., so I could get close to home by dark, and I'll keep in touch.

Caleb was going to come up over the weekend and you'd talked to Aaron earlier. He was busy with softball season coming to an end. You and Ken had tried to see Caleb on the way down, but he had gotten a call just before you got to Topeka. One meets children where they can. I remember meeting Nate on the side of a road to eat chicken between Topeka and Manhattan. We do what it takes to keep in touch; we can be happy that the kids are all busy and healthy.

October 10, 2006

You ended up spending eleven days in KC and boy were you ready to get home! It was a great weekend with a true fall—crisp, fresh, gorgeous colors, and not too cool.

Due to the blood clots, your chemo was on Monday night, so your schedule will change again. That's okay. The positive results will keep after it, full force. So glad we got the flowers in, since it is cooler now and rainy. You are looking really good. You have some puffiness yet, but you look so much better than when you were on more steroids.

Hopefully, you, Mom and I can get to Manhattan for a little shopping. Aaron has court today so everyone's thoughts are with him and Brennen. Your lab work looked pretty good yesterday. Steph's kids are so excited that Mr. Price will drive the bus this week. Evidently, the substitute never goes over thirty miles per hour, they were almost late for classes a couple times. I am cleaning closets, so I'd best get to it.

October 28, 2006

Man, time flies. I haven't been writing—I think because you're doing so well and things seem "normal." How wonderful! You had another chemo since I've last written. It went really well. You were home in five days. It is affecting your liver so they will have to try another drug combo; getting MRI again this time—fingers are crossed! You're doing great! You look good. You said you were feeling good, and your diet is more controllable. I am sure you have quirks and things we don't hear about, but I'm so glad things are going well.

Luke had his presentation and all is a go! Hard work pays off. He's so close to being done. We made some dough ornament recipe jars for the church bazaar; didn't take too long and they were really cute. Mom's started on her purse two or three times. You've started and I'm waiting on another skein to finish mine. It should be fun to see how they all come out. Our deadline of Christmas is fast approaching. Aunt Frances has passed away. Her services were lovely. Everyone was asking about you. It was a very difficult day, not only for the family, but also without you there.

We are going to a Halloween costume birthday party for Bruce Simmons and Evelyn Diederich tonight. We're going as M&M's. It should be fun and I hope our costumes still fit from a few years back. We got a new TV this week; a second one actually as the first one malfunctioned after a couple of days. We had to re-arrange furniture. I used to like to do that years ago. Now re-arranging everything takes too much thought and it is usually such a mess. I love the new TV, though. Addie found out she's one credit short on A&P for paramedic school. After twenty or so phone calls, she's enrolled in an online, eight-week course to be completed by January 1. So, she can still start her classes, otherwise it would be another year! Talk about someone having a couple of frustrating days—but it all worked out—$800.00 later, of course. Here's to a good week in KC and a good MRI report.

Shirley and Roger may come up next week; hope they get to see you. Mom's thinking about asking them to delay their trip until you're here. Kevin is working in Lincoln so it probably depends on that to some extent. After going to Oklahoma in such haste for the funeral, it will be nice to visit with them more.

October 31, 2006

You're on the way home today and called to let us know. Evidently, this chemo treatment is not working. The tumors are now larger than before and the MRI shows more tumor growth. The only word I can think of to describe how you feel is "devastated." We were all thinking you would have good MRI results. Well, we cry, we are upset, and question everything, BUT we need to go forward. Keep positive. You have spunk. You have desire and drive. You have Ken, the kids, and all of us. I met you and Ken at the folk's house. We all hugged, cried, talked, ate, discussed, and re-discussed. You have to be exhausted. All the kids were called. Now you and Ken need to rest, re-group and meet tomorrow, November 1, 2006, with clear eyes to search for more information and options.

November 1, 2006

I came out to your place after work. You're in better spirits and you have spent time on the Internet finding information regarding your situation. Tonight you start on your new oral chemo. Glad you have a chart! The amount of medicine you have to take is unbelievable. Ken came in after the bus route; the kids are glad he's back.

November 2, 2006

Mom made supper since Shirley and Roger are here. Kevin is working in Lincoln and so he also came down. It was a good evening. You're feeling good, and your pills are not making you sick. That is great! Hope it continues. We discussed a few options. Deb gave you info she'd run off on the computer. We talked about Houston, Mayo, California, and Mexico. Your steroids are four times what they were. Hopefully this will shrink the tumors enough that the chemo can destroy the cancer cells. This could work, you know. I've read on the Internet about how this does work in some patients when your earlier treatment didn't. I pray that this does work. On November 28 you go for another MRI. We will be holding our breath and have our fingers crossed. I am feeling some anger and I'm questioning—why you, my sister? You're so young, and you have so much to give. You have affected so many people in such a positive way. I'm so proud of you! We will fight this terrible disease with all we have. I'm determined you will be a survivor. I love you so much.

November 9, 2006

You, Mom, and I went shopping. You needed some clothes. You stayed in the dressing room with Mom, while I scoured the store looking for what you wanted, and something that would fit now, and later. This exhausted you. A few purchases were made, and before we went home, we decided to have a treat. We went to Famous Dave's. Nate was working and got to take a break. He sat with us for awhile. We all shared Famous Dave's delicious bread pudding—the best I have ever had. What a thrill to be able to do this. What a special moment it was.

We, (you, mom, and I) went to the Lady's Fair and the Tea House open house on Saturday. We enjoyed it all. Sometimes it was difficult, but, as troopers, we forged on. Lots of goodies, a beautiful day, and you were feeling really well. They cut your steroids down—not sure how much. You are going to have lab tests next week. You'd been doing well, came in for labs on November 8, and we were talking about making horseradish that evening when you had a sudden attack—pain in your chest, and difficulty breathing. It happened a couple times and wasn't subsiding. They took you upstairs, placed you on oxygen and ran tests. Your heart seems okay. Your doctor thinks it may have been a clot that dislodged, and you seem to be resting comfortably now. You will have a scan and hopefully the results will be available Thursday or Friday. You gave me and everyone quite a start, but at least you were in the right place for help and were not driving or by yourself! I called Ken, and he, of course, came right away. You were asleep when I left work, so didn't wake you.

We made about twelve jars of horseradish! I will stop in to see you tomorrow. Caleb came up to see you today and brought lots of goodies. Addie was here for a whirlwind overnight trip so she got to see you for a bit, too. Her financial aid was sent here, instead of KC, so she came to get it since she needed to pay her school expenses. She works weekends so she has a couple days off during the week. Nate had an evaluation last week at Famous Dave's and it went well. Aaron called to check on you. Clyde is no longer. It is hard to lose a dog, and of course, the kids are upset. Luke called earlier. You're waiting for callbacks from Mayo and Houston. Mom has progressed about two inches on her purse now. She has it down pat, after having to rip out numerous times. However, as I said, she's on a roll now. You and I are coming along fine with our projects, but I'm still waiting for my yarn delivery to finish the last inch. I finished the hats for Rahe, Addie and Hanna for Christmas. I'm addicted. I want to do one for mom for her birthday. All rims are a little different, but I still think I like yours the best. It's smaller and turned up just a bit. The girls will like the wider brims. Knitting has helped pass time when I'm up and can't sleep. Or when I'm worried about you. You always liked to knit, so I feel a connection with you when I knit. Crazy, huh? But, I do. Keith and Kyle are on their way to Arkansas to tear down a building and haul it back here to rebuild it—more energy than I have.

November 10, 2006

I went to Mom's after work. You and she were knitting your purses. You mostly watched her and the rest of us to see what we were doing. Your tests and scans were inconclusive. Guess that's good, since no problem was evident. You received an e-mail from Mayo regarding treatments. You seemed really tired today. You'd been up during the night and had quite a bit of nausea. The drugs are good, but they sure have a multitude of side effects.

November 25, 2006

Getting behind here, so will do a quick overview. You were anxiously awaiting the birth of the new grandbaby. He has arrived! Baby and mom are doing well. You and Ken had gone to Lincoln on Wednesday, November 15. Of course, the delivery was about two hours after you left. You both returned Thursday morning to see Trenton and hold him.

You and Mom made popcorn for PEO earlier, and you went there after the Lincoln trip. You were really tired. It would have made me tired, too. I called a couple times the past few days and you were doing pretty well. Your headaches seem better. You get relief when you sit up and are not lying down. You are sleeping a little better, however, not much though. I saw you in church November 19. It was an eventful week. You came out Monday and we had a very good visit. It was really a nice, crisp day. We talked about everything imaginable. It felt so good.

Caleb, Fran, and the kids came up on Tuesday and Wednesday to help around the house and yard. Caleb worked on Thanksgiving, and so they came to celebrate the holiday early. You said it seemed like they just flew doing work around the house, and you finally had to sit down and let them finish without you helping. Aaron, Jenny, and the kids came up for Thanksgiving at the folk's house. They enjoyed the day. Luke called. Addie, Caleb, Luke, and Sarah were all unable to be there due to work, but it was a good day. All the women went for a walk after dinner. It was a beautiful day, and you got a little winded, but were determined to walk around the entire block—and you did. No short cuts. There was some ball playing, football on the TV, lots of food, and a little knitting. This was the first day off your "diet" for chemo so you got some extras you weren't able to eat earlier. Addie and the new puppy, Sadie, came out to see you and Ken on Friday, November 24.

Saturday, Cindy and her family are coming. I hope that you will get some rest. You have lab here on Monday, and then you go to KC for your appointment on Tuesday. We all have our fingers crossed and have lost count of the prayers. GOOD NEWS is all we want. If not, well, we will go on to the next step if we have to.

We all went uptown on Friday night for the lighting of the Christmas lights. They served hot dogs, the stores were open, and there were people everywhere. They also had the tree auction. It was almost too much for you, but you wouldn't go home. Ken, however, couldn't get out of your sight or you'd get nervous. We all got so tickeled watching you and the puppy. I certainly hope I get a copy of the picture Delma Stamm took at her store. The pose was adorable. Sandi Brungardt asked about you. Glenda Sawin Stohs asked about you, too. Also, today at Casey's, Pat Hinkle asked about you. She had tears in her eyes and said that she prays for you every day. The girls and I went to Odell for a craft fair. Mom was not up to going. I got a couple items. Rahe likes to go, but Addie would rather have stayed home and worked on a puzzle. However, she did enjoy the food. Nate went back Friday afternoon for work, and the girls left tonight after supper. It was a good last few days, for everyone.

November 27, 2006

You looked really tired yesterday at church, and were having some balance issues. Ken helped by walking beside you and supporting you. It seemed like it was hurting you to walk. The steroids are making you have some puffiness, too. You were in for labs today and are doing better. I noticed Ken drove today, and I was not sure of the reason. The weather is damp, cold, and winter-like, so he probably just wanted to make sure you got here safe. You left after Ken got off his bus route to go to KC. Tomorrow is a huge day. You're having your MRI and will be able to see if this chemo is working. It's 2:00 a.m. and I can't sleep. I have had a headache off and on all night. I know it is tension. We all want good news tomorrow. I'm assuming you're up, too. May God bless you. Love, your sis.

November is over. It is now December.

December 3, 2006

The news wasn't what we wanted. The chemo is not working. Now, radiation is the next step. You have a consultation and I assume they will measure you for the mask you will wear during your treatments. Dr. Taylor got it set up in Manhattan. Dr. Reitz will be the oncologist there. At present, the schedule will be five days per week for six weeks. The tumors are twice the size they were. They have to reduce them and hopefully eradicate them. There are chances you take with this type of treatment. You have no choice. However, you have only a 10 percent chance of major problems. You are definitely having some difficulty. You're slower in your thought process. You tire easily, but who wouldn't? It's difficult for you to walk, and it hurts. A combination of things is causing it—disease, steroids, and arthritis. Yes, you're puffy, but that should get better. We're all upset, frustrated, and not sure what we can do to help you. Still, we have to keep positive, and keep your spirits up. You are allowed down time, BUT we then need to get you back to having a positive, up attitude—attitude, attitude, attitude.

I've been in the health field for thirty years (a tad more, actually) and people with a positive attitude always beat the odds and live longer, and we definitely want that. I saw Aaron and the family yesterday at the folk's house. They'd come to pick up their new dog at Keith and Deb's, and were hoping to see you and Ken. You and Ken had gone to Lincoln to see the new baby and to have supper with friends.

Today was gifts and goodies. I sure miss you. It seems you always were working somewhere or at least enjoying the festivities. It is just too much this year, plus, it is so cold. I went to Manhattan today with Mark. We met the kids for lunch, and got the Envoy back. Addie's car is repaired now. I got some different yarn to make you a splash hat. I finished it in a couple hours, but after it was done, I discovered it was a tad large. I decided to shrink it like crazy; otherwise, it wouldn't do you any good. Cross your fingers. I decided you needed some color and a little jazzy fun hat. It turned out great, and I can't wait to see it on you. It's late, and I need to get to bed.

December 12, 2006

Well, I lost track of time again. Your Christmas tree is decorated, compliments of Gracie and Jan. You didn't have any lab work last week. You went to see Dr. Reitz. The consultation was good and thorough. He had lots of information for you to read, and papers to sign. You look so good in that new hat! You went to Topeka after your consult and received a wig and head coverings. Caleb was able to come since he didn't have to work. All your boys are doing better now they know you and Ken are going for the radiation. Everyone just has to approach it as the next step. Dr. Reitz says he's pretty sure they will be able to get all the cancer. We are still not sure why they didn't do radiation earlier. I'm sure they have their reasons—only 10 percent chance of any permanent damage. You will lose your hair and it may not come back in front, but that's okay. We just want you better. Your wig looks nice and it's a good color for you.

I came to see you on December 9 for a while and we had lunch. We read information from Manhattan, and there was lots to absorb. I played bells at church today and then we all went to the annual turkey dinner. We all got to sit together. Mom and Dad even came. You seemed to enjoy yourself and you got to see lots of people you hadn't seen for awhile. The folks and Keith made it back from Oklahoma last night around 9:30 p.m. Aunt Dorothy's funeral was yesterday. Guess she got down to sixty pounds. I elected not to go and I stayed here with you. Keith represented us. They are all very concerned for you and prayers are being sent. There was ten inches of snow in Oklahoma City and it was snowing when they left Saturday night. Kansas was actually much nicer; imagine that! Robert was also unable to attend the services. It seems so strange to know both Frances and Dorothy are no longer going to be around. I know we all have limited time here, but we never really are prepared for losing loved ones.

I am going to meet you and Ken in Manhattan in the morning. I am curious as to what the doctors are doing, and they welcome family. We're planning to go to lunch. Then when you come back home, I am going on to KC to see the girls for a day. I will do some shopping, and see their house that's decorated for Christmas. I hope the weather holds until I get back. You know, my handwriting is outrageous. Sorry, but this does help me and hopefully it will help fill in some time gaps for you.

Ken put in a support bar for you in the bathroom, and he added a phone. Keith and Dad put in a high-rise stool that should make it easier for you. You are probably going to get more steroids, and we know your movement will be more difficult. You will be very tired due to radiation. Your radiation should be completed by the end of January, if all goes well.

December 11, 2006

I went to Manhattan with you and Ken. You were fitted for your face mask. You had either an x-ray or another scan. Ken and I are vague since you weren't sure what you'd have done. We went to lunch at Bob's Diner and then you went home to rest.

Ken came in earlier and was concerned about your various symptoms and that you needed help when getting up and down. I took him up to physical therapy and they helped him learn how to lift, etc. You and he had gone to look at Christmas lights last night and then went to eat. You couldn't get up out of the booth, and he called a friend to help. Well, there goes your outings for a while. You're too weak and you have difficulty thinking what to do. Caleb was presented his sergeant's badge Tuesday, but you were unable to go. This upset you terribly. Ken had gone to a funeral in Nebraska. You stayed home and rested. It is so difficult for you to get around.

After talking for a while today, we went for a walk outside. We were headed for the fire pit, but we only made it halfway! You stepped into a hole and fell. You know how to fall, and were not hurt. We tried and tried to get you up, but we couldn't. We got the giggles. I finally put a blanket under you, as the ground was damp. I called Mark to come help get you up. Ken was on the bus route and you wanted to get up "before Ken Price came home and saw you in this predicament." I don't know why, but you were really worried about that. After getting you in the house, we had tea, and then you rested. I left when Ken got home.

You were going to wrap some Christmas gifts. Deb, Pam and the folks came out later on.

You went to see Dr. Hodgson on Thursday. You are very confused again. You are tired; it is hard for you to get up, and you fall a lot. You had not been taking your glucose readings as routinely as needed. Your readings were 600 and 400 during the last few hours! Obviously, part of the confusion lays here. You could not remember if you took your pills or not, so now Ken is in total charge of your medications. You were given a choice of (1) staying home and letting Ken take care of you and minding him, (2) going to the hospital, or (3) going to the Homestead. You agreed to let Ken be in charge. I know it has to be extremely difficult, but it is the disease, not you.

Franklin and Van came up from Oklahoma. What a pleasant surprise. Mom and Dad had supper for everyone as they are leaving tomorrow morning. Van works at 7:00 tomorrow night. It was great to see them. You fell trying to get up the steps at Mom and Dad's. You were not hurt and the rest of the evening went well.

I went out Friday after work to check on you. You don't always answer the phone or sometimes cut the phone off unintentionally. Caleb, Fran, and the boys are here. You're in good hands and your glucose is now 200. You'd slept all morning and looked much better. Aaron called to see how things were. He'd talked to the folks earlier today. Guess he's tried to call you several times this week but got no answer. They are coming over tomorrow or Sunday. Keith suggested possibly getting flat-soled shoes for better stability. I think it is a great idea if we can just get you out of your shoes. Aaron thinks so too, and may get you new tennis shoes for Christmas. Everyone is planning to be at the folks for Christmas this year—the first time in ages. It should be fun and maybe we can get a group family picture. I wrapped gifts tonight and got ready for a progressive dinner party tomorrow. It should be lots of fun. We have the dessert. Time for bed. I'm tired. Prayers for you and family.

Did I mention Dad brought mistletoe from Oklahoma? Pretty cool stuff. It's the state flower, and I didn't know that. I stapled some to the archway on the deck and put some in a ribbon by the phone. Caleb brought you a pair of flat slippers. You were concerned about wearing them outside because of what people would think, but he said, ""Mom, you're losing your hair, why are you worried about what is on your feet?" You had no comeback on that, and now you are wearing the slippers.

December 21, 2006

It's the shortest day of the year.

So much has happened in such a short amount of time. It's been six days and you have undergone tremendous changes. I saw you Sunday, December 17, and I brought a bulletin to you and Ken as you couldn't attend church. It was the cantata and held at the Lutheran Church this year. Aaron, Jen, and the kids had gotten there about ten minutes before I did. You'd slept until noon and Ken got you up. You were confused about the day and the events from the last couple days. You are moving slower. Monday, December 18 was your first treatment and it went well. You returned here for your lab work to be done, and it was even harder for you to get around. Still, you are very tired. You thought you had eaten but you had not. Tuesday, Ken stopped by and was concerned about how to maneuver and lift you. You have fallen several times and it is difficult to get you up. He is checking into a lift. I went out after work while Ken was on his bus route. You were just sitting in the bathroom. You had forgotten how long you had been there. Since you have a urinary tract infection, it adds to your other problems. When it rains, it pours. You are so very tired; you just wanted to go to bed and were out as soon as your head hit the pillow.

Mom and I took you to radiation on Wednesday. It was raining. It is so nice to have two people so there is always someone with you. I parked the car and went to get it, while mom was with you. We got you into the office but ended up using a wheelchair since you were weak and your legs weren't strong enough to support you. You had a headache earlier. After treatment, Dr. Reitz saw you and visited about twenty minutes with us all. He was so impressed when we told him you had been not only the CEO of the KSDS, Inc., but had been there since its' inception. He knew of the facility and its cause.

We took you to get your wig trimmed. It is so difficult for you to get in and out of the vehicle. Megan, the hairdresser, came out to you! She put the wig on you, saw how it needed to be shaped, and then she put it on another customer who was in the shop and cut it. She then came back out to see how it fit you. She would not take a dime for doing it. The wig looks great on you. It must have been comfortable, as you left it on the rest of the day.

You slept in the afternoon, as you were exhausted. We had written down everything that was told to us at the doctor's office and gave the info to Ken. He has a notebook where he records everything, so he can keep track of all the details.

Today, I came out early so Ken could go on the bus route. We're not to leave you alone in case you would fall or have a seizure. Sometimes, you have no strength to get up and the next minute you do. You are using a walker and it does seem to help support you. Your balance is off. Guess you were agitated today at radiation. It took longer to do but you eventually got your treatment. They had Ken come back to help calm you. In addition to all your drugs, you now have antibiotics for your urinary tract infection and a pill to calm you down so you are not so anxious and nervous.

They seem to think you are showing some signs of depression. HELLO—who wouldn't? I went to see you after work, and Dad went with Ken today. You hadn't slept and you weren't talkative at all. You appeared to have a headache but you said it's okay and didn't want anything for it. We need to keep forcing you to drink water. It is hard for you to sit still or get comfortable. One feels so helpless since we can't help you. It is so frustrating, and I get so angry and question why. I'm still trying to find a cause or reason for this. I know there probably will not be an answer.

December 22, 2006

Mom went with Ken today and you had a good day there. You were smiling today and moving a tad better. Oh, mom's purse is done! I'm still waiting for my yarn. Can you believe she is the first one done? She didn't even knit before this! Bob King offered to help where needed.

December 25, 2006

Merry Christmas.

I saw you yesterday. Rahe, Addie, and I came to see you and Ken after church. Luke had come home, and you'd had family Christmas with Ken's side of the family on Saturday. I noticed you'd slowed down some but were alert and talking.

On Thursday, you were tired and not talkative at all. Your glucose is still elevated.

Now it's Christmas. Everyone is here except Sarah; she left at 10:00 for work. It was a very full day with lots of food. You had great difficulty with weakness in your legs. You knew what was going on, though. Ken offered the prayer. You were first in line, but not because you wanted to be. Luke helped select the correct foods to try to get your glucose down. He plans to talk to Reitz and Hodgson regarding your care and he wants to get a dietician out for some counseling. Lots of pictures were taken. Santa and Mrs. Santa visited. Presents were opened. You were number one in our gift exchange, and even though you had last choice and could take any present you wanted, you "kept" your gift. The gift you gave this year was a cookbook from Paula Dean. Pam got that. You love Paula Dean.

Everyone is getting ready to leave as they either have to go home or on to more Christmas dinners. You were tired and wanted a nap. There was a lot of commotion going on, and you were so tired. It was wonderful having family together today—so very special. All your kids and grandkids were here. We took group pictures and Dad kept saying, "Take just one more." I am anxious to get them back. Delma Stamm had taken the picture at Thanksgiving of you in your hat and holding Addie's puppy, Sadie. It is adorable; I'll make copies for everyone. It was a good weekend and tomorrow you start radiation again. There will be no rest until you are done. Five treatments down, and twenty-five to go.

Week of December 25

Luke went to radiation with you this week. It takes two now, and we don't leave you alone. This leaves someone with you as the other person does other necessary things. Dad, Aaron, Mom, and I are taking turns. Caleb comes up from Topeka when he is off.

The ramp is up at your house. Ken bought it never thinking you'd be the one needing it. Life takes many surprising and unanticipated turns. You wanted your home to be accessible for anyone physically impaired, and now you are the one benefiting from it.

You are very dehydrated. It is hard to get you to drink and your glucose is very high. Everyone is trying to get you to drink more water and eat better foods. You are not feeling hungry and food tastes different due to chemo and radiation. You had IV's for hydration towards the end of the week. You're drinking better. You have lost twenty-five pounds. You say you don't notice, but we do. Steroids still make you puffy. However, you are better. Some days you are more alert. This is an exhausting ordeal and your body needs rest.

Luke helped Ken with your diet. Ken doesn't really like to cook, and having to prepare for a special diet just makes it more difficult. Luke went through all the food and pitched anything that was deemed not good for you. He cleaned some, too. Of course, he also did a few puzzles while he was here. He came out one night when Nate was here and it was really great seeing him. We caught up on his progress of finishing school and getting ready for the next chapter of his life. The weekend of December 29, 30, and 31 was rainy and then snowy. It was a good stay-at-home weekend. You got lots of needed rest. You can walk on your own fairly well and you use the walker for support if walking around the house for your exercise. The bathroom is quite a chore. You have difficulty getting there and back, but so far, and somehow, you do.

January 1, 2007

HAPPY NEW YEAR!

We went out for a while. You were in good spirits and actually started some conversation. You even wanted to have some tea. We watched out the front window as Aaron and Ken put the railing up for the ramp. You're ready now. Today you spoke a little about your feelings. Wonderful! We all know that parts of this disease process are so humiliating. We, however, are looking at the big picture. You smile more and are quicker in response, both verbal and through your facial expressions. You appear to enjoy some quiet time. I always turn the TV off when just you and I are here. Your hearing is very sensitive.

Ken's friend, and mentor, gave you a baby monitor to use so if Ken is in another room he can hear if you need assistance. You commented you weren't looking forward to the upcoming trips to Manhattan. Mom and Dad came out as Aaron and I were leaving. I'd prepared some meals, so all Ken needs to do is take them out and heat them up if needed, and you're ready to eat. If this helps, I will continue to do it. If not, I will try a different route. I subscribed to a diabetic menu site for a month. I plugged in your info and it gave a month's worth of meals, a grocery list and calorie count, etc. I hope it works.

Well, the Christmas decorations are down and we're ready for a new year. Here's to a great one; one that finds you healthier and your spirit alive and well. Prayers, and God bless you.

I often think of our piano playing days—such great memories. I hope in the future if we can't play together, we will remember. You will always be beside me on the bench—if only in thought, as I hope I am for you.

January 3, 2007

Dad and Ken took you to treatment yesterday. I came out in the afternoon so Ken could run some errands. You were up, in good spirits, joined in the conversation, and asked for something to drink. Hot tea was your choice. How wonderful. You visited well and your glucose is below 400 again. You are a tad restless as you wanted to get into a different position but it was difficult. You got tired after about an hour and went in for a nap. You walked well.

Today, Aaron and I took you to treatment, and Caleb met us. You did great and we were back in good time. It was so hilarious. Ken's car was gone when we got back and we all thought he was gone. However, when we made a turn to get in front of the ramp, there was Ken—in the hot tub! We were so surprised that we all just burst out laughing—even you. I don't know who was more surprised, him, or us. I am sure it had been a while since he'd been able to enjoy that so we hated that we had interrupted him. It makes for a great story, though, and oh, to hear you giggle and laugh—how can I describe that?

You are very picky about your food. Ken isn't giving you anything that Luke didn't have on the list. So, I guess I will forget the diabetic diet. It makes it easier for Ken and hopefully you'll get better at eating. Lunch didn't set well with you today. I just about lost Aaron when you got sick, but then you were fine. Aaron came back in the room. I filed your nails and gave you a mini hand massage with some lotion Rahe sent you. I left, and then Aaron was going to clean out your car and help Ken do some things. You were ready for your well-deserved nap. You are improving—gradually. We are all so excited. You're getting some spunk in you, and boy, your facial expressions leave no doubt about what you are thinking.

January 10, 2007

It's been one week and so many things have happened. You seem to continue to improve, and you actually start conversations. You are requesting things like hot tea, something to drink, or you tell us if you want different places to sit.

Jan Taylor went with you on Thursday. You had trouble with your legs supporting you last night. The folks came out to help Ken, and to help with getting you out of bed. You were in Manhattan and went down again. You went down again at home. Jan realized just how ill you are. I think it was quite difficult for her. So many people just have no idea how ill you really are, even though we tell them. It is very difficult for us to explain and for them to grasp and accept it. Ken called Dad to come help you up. When Dad got there he said, "What are you doing down there?" and you replied, "Waiting on you." That was so funny. They finally got you in bed. I went out after work and you're better. Radiation is absolutely zapping your energy and you have little muscle tone in your legs for support. The family ordered a mini-pedal cycle for you while you sit on the couch. Terry Taylor went with Ken and you on Friday and it was a better day. You rested during the weekend and are doing well. On Sunday, Pastor Phil came out and gave you communion. That meant so much. You were feeling good and even asked to sit on the regular couch. You walked well. You wanted your wig on and I could see your effort in trying to make "normal" conversation as if everything was "normal."

Caleb came up Monday and Tuesday. After your Wednesday appointment, he went back to Topeka. He had court, but he's planning to meet you on Thursday again. He will come back again on Saturday. You had a horrible headache today and couldn't shake it. You couldn't get comfortable. You had trouble drinking and seemed to choke a lot. You were very tired and didn't want to eat when you got home. You just wanted a nap.

Aaron and I came over today. It helps to break up the drive for Ken. Dad is good about going almost every day. Mom wants to help more but is not strong enough. It is difficult for her not going along more. I think Lila, Deb, or Michelle may come out while Ken does the bus route today. He's only doing afternoon routes and it seems to work well.

Everyone knows you don't like medicines but you may need to start taking more pain medicine. It will help take the edge off, at least. We just don't like seeing you in pain and not able to help you control it. You have lost thirty-six pounds. The girls at Reitz's office showed us your treatment room today. Gretchen Oehmke works there and it is so comforting to know someone there. All the staff is very accommodating. Seeing all the computers and the actual machine that is used for treatment is amazing. Science has come so far and yet has so far to go. Oh, you get to keep your mask. Wow, not sure if that makes a person happy or not, but you paid a pretty penny for it. You might as well keep it—put it in your room and put your wig on it or use it as a hat stand. You are pretty much in a wheelchair now when out of the house. No one wants to risk you falling or breaking a bone.

January 15, 2007

Last Thursday and Friday, you did really well. Your legs were weak but your thought process is improving. The weekend brought some snow, a little sleet and it was very cold. It is one degree outside. Wind is also present. This is a good time to stay in and keep warm. You are exhausted and your legs are like noodles. At your appointment on Monday, Dr. Reitz discussed concern for your safety, since you are fully dependent on someone for everything, due to being so weak. He suggests some help—as in twenty-four-hour care. Ken and you visited regarding this and Ken phoned your boys. They agreed if you were in favor of it. If it is best for you, then it is a go. It is temporary only. When you get done with radiation and physical therapy at the hospital, you'll be strong enough and independent enough to go home. Actually, Karen, you spent time in KC during chemo like this and at least here, you will have visitors and be accessible to family and friends more readily. In addition, since I work here, I'll bebop in to see you often. If you need something during the day, I can help.

You have nine days of treatment left now. When you return tomorrow following treatment, they will admit you into the hospital for care. They are planning to put you in a room in the east hallway where it isn't so noisy. We'll get your room fixed up for you with personal stuff and make it feel homey. The hospital has good staff and I'm sure you will be treated very well. Your family will be free to come and go as they want.

Caleb came up again this week. Aaron's coming over, too. Luke offered to help pay expenses but Ken assured him you have enough to cover costs. I came to see you today and Jan Matlack came for a visit. You drank like three-and-one-half glasses of water. I am so glad you're finally drinking fluids. You look good and are wearing hats a lot—you look cute in a hat. You have always looked good in hats. Mom's birthday was yesterday and you remembered. Still, however, you get confused about what day it is and whether something has happened today or yesterday. You are getting better in thought. Sometimes I think you are afraid to say something in case you are wrong. If you use a straw, you don't have as much difficulty swallowing and choking. They lowered your steroids today and if all goes well, they will lower them again next week. You are getting tired of one position but it's often hard to find one that is comfortable. You have some discomfort in your rib areas. I think it is due to lifting you with bear-hug-like transfers.

January 21, 2007

You went into Intermediate Care Swing Bed at the hospital on Tuesday. Dr. Reitz felt it was safer to have you there and it is much easier to maneuver you. No one at the hospital can believe the family was still taking care of you at home. If not for Dad and Ken, you would have been here earlier. It is very difficult for everyone but it seems to be working out well.

Your routine is usually to get up early and have physical therapy around 7:00 to 7:30, eat breakfast, and get ready for the Manhattan trip. You will have more physical therapy when you return. Then lunch is served and you get to take a well-deserved nap. You are up again around 3:30 to 4:00. Supper is at 5:30. You are usually ready for bed around 7:00 p.m. You are exhausted by that time. You have only five days left of radiation and I know you can't wait for this treatment to be over. Ken had the flu today so the folks and I took turns being with you. We had five inches of snow, but no ice. You are getting stronger. You can lift your legs some and your arms seem stronger. Today you combed your hair, did your own mouth care, glossed your lips, and poured your own water, while holding the pitcher and the glass. You drank from a glass more instead of using a straw. I am trying to keep your nails up for you. They seem to grow so fast. It must be due to the protein drinks you're getting. Sarah sent some nice lotion to you and you've been using that. Everyone here loves the smell of it and it works well, too. Your hands are so soft.

January 22, 2007

Dad and I are taking you for radiation tomorrow. Nate is going to help in transferring you. His Monday class doesn't start until 10:30 so it should work great.

Dad and I got you in the car at the hospital and tried to put the wheelchair in the trunk, but the chair decided to take flight! Dad ran after it before it ran into a car or into the street. He is actually quite speedy. Quite the sight we were. Finally, we were on our way. You were probably wondering "What next?" You seem to be looking at everything on the way down. You don't talk much, but want to sit up and look out. You want no pillow for your head and nothing to drink. Nate met us there and we got you inside for treatment. You were having difficulty breathing. After your treatment, the doctor decided to do another scan to rule out possible blood clots and he said it could take a while. They may even keep you in Manhattan. Although Nate was reluctant to do so, he went to class. The scan is negative and we return home. You have four treatments left.

Aaron is driving tomorrow. Luke e-mailed today and he talked to Ken. He so wishes he could do more. You've had a couple headaches this week and tonight you had terrible lower leg pain. It is hard for you to get comfortable. We can't wait for the end of radiation so your body can begin to "normalize."

Peggy L. Chapin

The swelling should start to go down. They may decrease your steroids this week.

Another MRI is scheduled for February 23. Consultation with the doctor will follow and I'm not sure if they have a date for that yet. Ken is ready to get you back home and I'm sure you're ready, too. The folks got the family Christmas picture back. They had Sarah inserted into the picture. We showed you the picture and you seemed to understand what it was all about. I sent some of our family pictures off for prints. Our immediate family will change after June. Everyone is getting excited. Rahe's baby is due June 11. Her name is Isabella. We are going to KC this weekend to celebrate Rahe's birthday and clean carpets. Sounds like a fun time, no?

January 23, 2007

Aaron and Ken took you to Manhattan today. It was not a good day. You were having such difficulty breathing. They put oxygen on you for a while and it seemed to help. Meanwhile, Ken was in with the doctor and upon completion of that visit, Ken came to the waiting room and took Aaron outside for a review of your status.

The doctor feels that physical therapy is too much for you. Therefore, you need to either cut back or discontinue it. He feels the radiation is not working. However, he assured the family that had you not had the radiation, you would not have lasted this long. His suggestion—comfort and care.

You are unable to communicate well. You appear to be in a state of fog and are distant. The ride home was agonizing. The family has been informed. The hours keep going by and no one is sure what the next step will be.

We sit with you. They have some meds to help you. It is hard to go home, to rest, and leave you here.

Sunday, you had asked twice to go home. Later, Mom wondered which home you were talking about.

January 24, 2007

It is 1:30 a.m. I awakened from a dream, for lack of better terms. It was so real. I was reliving our last communion. I could have touched you; everything was exactly as it was then. All I could keep thinking about was you having difficulty breathing. After a short while, I just got up, got ready for work (as I was the early person the next day), and came to spend the rest of the night with you. I am so glad I did. The night for you was restless. You could not find a comfortable position. You couldn't rest. We kept asking if you were in pain, but you said, "No." Still, you kept holding your head and would touch your chest. You said you felt pain in your legs and we could not get the pain to stop. You couldn't swallow without difficulty. You were thirsty. You begin choking around 3:30 to 4:00. Suctioning helped. I called Ken and he came in. You seemed to rest a little easier. I did go to work around 7:00 a.m. Caleb had come up the night before (and got a warning for speeding—eight miles over). We all got a chuckle over that.

I couldn't stay out of your room so I finally just clocked out. Thank goodness for Steph and Evelyn. They have been so understanding and supportive throughout this entire ordeal. The folks were here most of the day, too. The decision was made to forgo radiation treatment. You are too weak. Instead, you are on cocktails—morphine and a pain patch. You are finally getting comfortable. You won't eat. You do not want a drink. You have no desire, and no strength. They gave you an IV for hydration. Keith and Deb came here to see you. Aaron is back.

Cloud County Community College had a bomb threat and the entire college was closed down and waiting on the bomb squad to arrive. Aaron's family is coming over. Craig, Andrea, and Trenton are here. Luke is getting things lined up so he can be on his way. Ken is wonderful—so loving, caring—yet so beside himself as not wanting you to suffer but he doesn't want to lose you. None of us do.

Caleb spent tonight with you. He will call if anything changes.

January 25, 2007

We got a call at 3:00 a.m. Everyone was told it did not look good. Luke left from Oklahoma City. The rest of us went to the hospital—a vigil, if you like. We are so in hope that Luke gets here and he is safe during his travels—so far away and yet not.

Your breathing was again altered. It was difficult to hear you, but no one wanted to leave. It was a long, yet short night. You had no responses. There was no movement of your arms or legs. You were not able to speak, and rarely did we think we saw any movement, somewhere.

Luke got to Concordia and picked up Jenny. We were all thinking, "Please get here." Within five miles of Washington, Luke was stopped and given a warning ticket for speeding. Upon hearing who he was, and the situation, he was told to go on. Finally, at 9:40 in the morning, Luke arrived. Everyone left the room so your boys and Ken had time alone with you. Your breathing changed again. You were more at ease. It is was if you were waiting for Luke to get here.

Eventually, we all came back in. Mark left for work. I was to call him. Keith came back. We were around your bed. I rubbed your arm and held your hand. Ken had stepped out to make a phone call. Your eyes began to open ...slowly. I told everyone, "Look, Karen is awake. She is awake. She is here. Karen is back!" Ken came back into the room.

We gathered around you. Your eyes were open. You see, you—Karen—are here. You are in that moment, "you," before these last months of altering life changes. You have a tear; you are emitting love and a feeling of peace. You cross over; you have passed on to life with God. We grieve, and we cry. We don't want to lose you—there is grieving, and yet also a sense of peace and comfort. We have let you go. Never have I experienced such emotion. It is beyond explanation. May all our lives on earth be as yours in the end.

One need not be afraid of death. There is a heaven.

Time of death on earth, 10:23 a.m., Thursday, January 25, 2007.

* * *

I have put the last page of this journal in the form of a letter to Karen. It just seemed to be what I needed to do.

Journal entry for January 25, 2007

Karen,

It was to be your last week of radiation. You were to get better. The cancer was to be gone. We had been assured that had you not taken radiation, we would have lost you sooner.

In the end, you were given what is referred to as cocktails—morphine and pain patches. You were given "comfort and care." Your family was there. You had waited for Luke to arrive. Everyone had time with you. You were being talked to and touched. Then, your eyes began to open. It was almost as if in slow motion. Then you—Karen—your whole being was there. You were, in that moment—you—the Karen before these last months of altering life changes. You knew we were there. You had a tear. You emitted love and a feeling of peace. Then (as is often said) in the blink of an eye, you passed on to a life with God.

We grieve, and we cry out your name. We don't want to lose you, but now we are the ones who feel a peace, calm, and are comforted. It is euphoric. We have let you go.

May all our lives on earth be as yours in the end. One need not be afraid of death. There is a heaven—another world. God is absolute.

Your faith was strong. Your life was an abundance of love.

Family—it has changed. It will continue to change, but our family will always encompass you.

We love you, Karen. May it have been said and showed enough.

Your spirit will be with us all forever. Until we are reunited with you again, you have our blessings of peace and eternal love.

Love always, your sister, Peg

* * *

In the days after Karen's passing, I still felt the need to write in her journal. It was a habit of the last few months, I guess. Therefore, I wrote down words that represent things done, words of things remembered, and just words of things.

The grieving starts.
Prayer for Karen
Final goodbyes
Mortuary
Arrangements
A visit to the grave site
Meals are brought in
Pictures bring back memories
Family
Friends
Lists and things to do, things done, and things requested
More food
Phone calls
Hugs
Tears
Laughter
Memories
Thank you's
Going through motions
Hunt for personal memorabilia
Togetherness
Services
Scriptures
Tears
Paper products
Meals
Decisions
Restlessness
Comfort
Sharing

Tenseness
Grandchildren
Cousins
Aunts
Uncles
Siblings
Parents
Friends
Cards
Flowers
Memorials
Music
Strength
Your day
Inurnment
Cold, crisp, clear
Sunshine
Simple
Elegant
Sorrow
Tears
Comfort
Peace
Presence of the Holy Spirit
Church
People everywhere
Over 500 attend services
Song
Piano Music
Eulogy
Video
Expressions of sympathy
Hugs
Tears
Flowers—sorting, sharing, and delivery to gravesite

Another speeding warning—Nate—on the way home from
the cemetery
Strength
Courage
Pride
Humbleness
Acceptance
Clouds
Exhaustion
Finality
Looking back
Moving forward
So many lives, touched forever
Pass it on
A part of Karen is with us forever in our hearts

As Karen said,
"If you are going to do something, do it right."
And, she did.